TABLE OF CONTENT

This book is divided into SEVEN sections:

1. Role of a bedside Nurse: Know Who, What, Which, and When

2. Teamwork: Customer service/ CQI

3. Leadership Role and Nursing Instructors: Clinical and Classroom

4. Comics: Do Nurses have sense for humor

5. Bullies: Bullies in the work place

6. CQI Continuous quality improvement

7. The Emotional aspect of Nursing

"The very first requirement in a hospital is that it should do the sick no harm.

"To understand God's thoughts, we must study statistics; for these are the measures of his purpose."

There is no part of my life upon which I can look without pain."

"The amount of relief and comfort experienced by the sick has been carefully washed and dried, is one of the commonest observations made at a sick bed."

-Florence Nightingale

CHAPTER ONE:

THE ROLE OF A BEDSIDE NURSE: WHO, WHAT, WHICH, WHY.

Let me just begin by saying that as a Registered Nurse, you must assess, diagnose, plan, influence, organize, and be able to control the outcome of your patient care.

"Good morning Jenny, it is 07:00AM. Can I get a report on Mr. Sg in Room 202, and do you also have room 201, 203, 205, and 217?" Once you come to work in any unit, you clock in at the right time per hospital policy, check the assignment and find out the patient assigned to you. After all of this, you receive your report. It is recommended that you go from room to room during the report to prevent blame, in other words, you are able to observe your patient while the outgoing nurse is still around in case you need some clarifications in the report given. SBAR is any effective communication process in which we use during report and communicating with the physician.

Let me know when you are ready and I will give you report on those patients, but I do not have room 217, I believe Jackie has room 217. Who is the Charge Nurse in your shift? Why and what is the problem? I do not know why she assigned room 217 to me since it's a long walk. Well, I think that particular room is in the Isolation room. She is only trying to be fair in the distribution of the isolation rooms so that one nurse will not have all the isolation rooms. Okay, that makes a lot of sense. Is the consent for **PICC line** placement signed for Mr. SG in room 202? Yes, consent has been signed and is in the chart. Also, room 203 was complaining of chest pain earlier today, so they were given 3 doses of nitroglycerine, EKG and cardiac enzyme level **to be done.** Every 6-8 hours for 24 hours, please follow up on that. The determination for excellent nursing care delivery system on a medical/surgical floor should be based on the following criteria:

1. Patient satisfaction
2. High standards of care
3. Support from other Healthcare workers
4. How equal and fair the assignment for all Nursing staff is

5. Job satisfaction and the relation with staff morale
6. Role confusion and poor communication
7. Patient care activities and outcomes
8. Avoiding too much bureaucracy in Nursing

Difficult assignments should be identified and be equally distributed among the staff. Sometimes, it is difficult to pre-determine the acuity for the patient to the floor. Resignation should be minimized and staff morale should be uplifted.

If you are able to see the things that other people do not see, you automatically become their messiah, a trailblazer, a pacesetter, and a pathfinder. When you are able to find a solution to the problem and you are not afraid of the unknown, you are being proactive. You take action and do things that others dread. People will want to be a part of you. They will want to join you. When people depend on you for direction, it commands respect. In nursing, when you do a good job, people will notice this and have confidence in your judgment; this leads to trust.

CHAPTER TWO:

TEAMWORK
CUSTOMER SERVICE.

WHO IS MY CUSTOMER?

TEAM : STANDS FOR;

T : TOGETHER

E : EACH OTHER

A : ACCOMPLISH

M : MORE

When we work together, we accomplish more. Let us motivate, encourage and empower each other because the goal is quality improvement of the hospital.

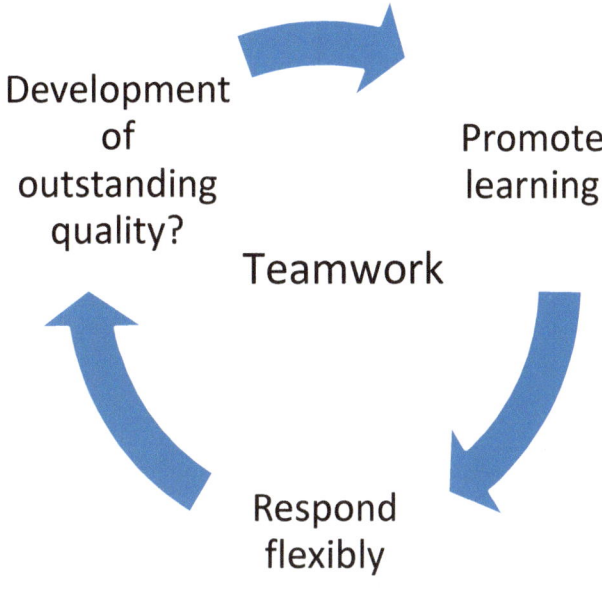

In healthcare, we continuously work on projects to improve the quality of the health of the community we serve. Sandra, what continuous quality improvement (CQI) is your team working on this quarter? CQI is the development of a process to ensure that programs are intentionally designed and systematically in place. CQI is also referred to as performance and quality improvement. We are working on customer service. Customer service is the new way of marketing personal service to the public. Courtesy and service are the emphasis on merchandising today and it applies to the employees who are working directly to the public. They serve more than just the employer. Customer service is an important part of the job and should not be neglected or put aside.

The most vital asset of a company is the customer. The Joint commission on Accreditation on Healthcare Organization (JCAHO) announced its Agenda for change in 1986. They have stated that the "philosophical context for the Agenda of Change is embedded in continuous quality improvement."

Let your light shine before men so that they may see your good works and glorify your Father which is in heaven. Matthew 5:16

A great customer service skill is the key. It is the provision of excellent service to your customer before, during, and after service. According to Turban et al (2002), customer service is a series of activities designed to enhance the level of customer satisfaction - the conscious feeling that a product or service has met the customer's expectations. The perception of success of such interactions will be dependent on employees "who can adjust themselves to the personality of the guest." – Micah Solomon

Please explain to me again, how we can provide an unforgettable customer experience. These are basic guidelines for good customer service.

1. Be a good listener: listen carefully to your customers
2. Learn and know your customers' what, who, and why.

3. Anticipate your customer needs (patients, Patients' families, visitors, and your colleagues)
4. Personalize it, make it your personal responsibility
5. Be there and available for your customer
6. Be effective and efficient and respond quickly to their needs
7. Demonstrate appreciation and follow up with your customers to make sure that their needs are met.
8. Be knowledgeable and creative. Give your customers something positive to remember and say about you.
9. Increase your job satisfaction by improving your skills. Attend training sections and learn from co-workers.
10. Adopt a supportive attitude, be part of the solution and do not point fingers. Play a

positive role and speak up when necessary. Never ignore a problem.

In nursing, we are full of determination and desire to achieve our goals, we have definiteness of our purpose and have persistent effort of working on our desired goal for ten, twenty, twenty-five, thirty and sometimes, thirty-five years.

"You are the salt of the earth and the light of the world and you are here to shine for the sick and their families."

Sometimes, our desires are able to survive pain, disappointment, disbelief, shock, discouragement, defeat, criticism, and constant nagging from your supervisor or your colleagues. But most often, we are quiet and look somewhere else where the grasses are greener (probably), success has many parents, but failure is an orphan. Wealth maketh many friends, but the poor is separated from his neighbors. Prosperity does not come by crooked men, but by faithfulness, successful people are determined and understand the value of persistence. Without persistence, there will be no achievement of success.

Congratulations for being a Nurse. You are in a noble profession. Love nursing and nursing will love you back. Nurses are among the line job personnel in hospital. The nurse managers, nurses, and unit coordinators are among the core for the organization. It is therefore important to lead by examples and be a team player. Always remember teamwork is the key to success and a great element for a good shift. There is no single individual with sufficient experience, ability education, academic excellence and knowledge to ensure the accumulation of a great work without the cooperation of other people (physicians, nurses, physical therapist, occupation therapist, speech therapist, and respiratory therapist). There are certain things that are not nursing: procrastination, passing the buck all the time, blaming others for your mistakes, feeling indifferent and irresponsible behavior.

Nurses are generally honest, kind, compassionate, caring, knowledgeable, educated leaders and motivators who are also great listeners. We like to lead and demonstrate our knowledge and capabilities. We are not afraid of constructive criticism. Nurses always have the desire to succeed in life. On reflection therefore, it is clear that there is a growing need for a role transition for the new nurses and for new nurses to benefit from the experience and leadership of the seasoned nurses.

CHAPTER THREE: COMICS: DO NURSES HAVE SENSE OF HUMOR, WHILE MAKING SENSE.

As we all know, "the only way to get through life is to laugh through it. You either have to laugh or cry. I prefer to laugh."- Marjorie Pay Hinckley

Nurses also like to laugh so they talk crazy shit on their break time with the right people, at the right place and the right time for the right reasons. We call it recipes for "stress reduction".

Velvet walked into the break room and said, "I am off tomorrow and will be at 7-Eleven all day. I am open for business for 24 hours at the store with my husband." She enjoys talking about intimacy with her husband. Very entertaining. Please keep your questions and answers to yourself. Ten minutes later, Jessica walked in the break room "My patient in room 213 hemoglobin level is 7.8/21.4, he is symptomatic, feels very dizzy, and his blood pressure is 102/56. I called the doctor and I am waiting for a call back and possible transfusion of PRBC, consent, a type and cross match is needed before transfusion."

"I think you should encourage your patient to remain in bed, give him the urinal, instruct him not to get out of bed. What is his oxygen saturation at this time? Does he need supplemental oxygen at this time? Place the bed alarm on because we do not want him to fall since he is light headed. As good team players, we communicate our concerns and discuss with each other before calling the doctor. The doctors like it when you know what you are doing. Especially the trauma doctors as they want competent nurses. Oh, I forgot to tell the charge nurse that the lab called and said that patient is positive for **MRSA of the right and left nare and in his right foot wound.** So, the patient is now on contact isolation/precautions. As a healthcare worker, it is very important to approach all body fluids including blood, urine, etc as if they are contagious from the beginning. Do not take chances. We often discovered out that patients are contagious after taking care of them for a while.

It is important to be safe than sorry so that at the end.

What is MRSA? Methicillin-Resistant Staphylococcus Aureus.

Some for the common risk factors that could lead to MRSA in a chronic wound are;

    Patient is transferred from a long-term care facility such as nursing homes, long-term antibiotics, recent incarceration and overcrowded space, recent hospitalization.

"Patients with a chronic wound positive for MRSA may be carrying the microorganism in multiple body sites including the nose, rectum, perineum or axillary, percutaneous line insertion sites, tube feeding, as well as indwelling

catheter" (CHRONIC WOUND CARE-The essentials page, 107).

The right intravenous antibiotic is ordered by the doctor and the level for the antibiotic monitored percutaneous lines discontinued. Consultation for infectious disease doctor implemented and patient condition monitored.

Like I said earlier, Bedside Nurses have some comics or joke-moments while we suffer.

Here is another comic for nurses. Four nurses died and went to heaven where they met St. Peter at the gate of heaven. He asked the first nurse, "What did you do while you were on Earth?" She replied, I was a nurse in a comic hospital, took care of the sick, married, had children and raised my children to be responsible adults. I also took care of my sick husband but did not have time for myself." St. Peter replied, "You did a good job but next time, take care of yourself before taking care of others, enter the kingdom of heaven." Then came the second nurse and he asked, "What role did you play on Earth?" She replied "I did the same that the other nurse did, except I did it while I was in Australia. I had to work my rear end off." St. Peter replied "You should also enter the kingdom of heaven," and she entered happy and excited. The third nurse came in and St. Peter asked, "What did you do on Earth?" and she replied, "I worked in a male prison, took care of various hard core criminals and also married a miserable husband, took care of him for 35 years. He came home every night drunk and he constantly cheated on and abused me." St. Peter replied, "Noble woman, you had more rough days on Earth than anybody else, enter the kingdom of heaven and I will send the angel to wash and feed you." St. Peter asked, "Why didn't you dump that loser? For better or worse does not mean hell." Then came the fourth nurse and St. Peter asked her, "So what did you do on Earth?" She replied, "I did not do much, I was just an HMO nurse. I enjoyed my life on Earth and made sure that everybody with HMO went through their doctor for referral even if they were about to die." St. Peter hesitated and said, "I thought about leaving you in heaven for only three days, but I changed my mind. Hell is the best place for you." The nurse replied, "Please send me to heaven with my colleagues so that we can share our life experiences together." St. Peter replied, "While you were having fun on Earth, they were working very hard. It is payback time, you reap what you sow."

Inside the Elevator

A nurse coming in to work met a nine-year old body in the elevator. He said, "My mom is in the second floor, she just had a baby girl." Today is the happiest day of my life. I am going to be his only brother for the rest of my life." The nurse replied, "Congratulations, but what did your mom tell you about talking to a stranger?" "I was told not to talk to strangers, but you aren't a stranger, you're a nurse", the boy said.
"What is my name?"
Boy: "Your name is nurse and you work here."
Nurse: "How do you know that I work here? Try to be safe and always have an adult you can trust around next time. Have a nice day." It is another day in the break room with the right people, the

right audience, the right time, and the right reasons.

Nurses Vacation

Dolly: "I will be going on vacation with my husband; we have not had a vacation for a long time."
Shelby: "Have a good vacation, and make sure that the girls are properly taken care of."
Dolly: "What girls? What are you talking about my husband? I am going to stop been your friend if you continue to talk about landscape and girls. We are Muslims and what you just said is against our religion."
Dolly's marriage was arranged so she does not understand all the nicknames given to all our body parts.

Clueless Doctors

Most of the time, the doctors have no idea what we do and could be careless about our function. Some of them see us as object that can be manipulated and relegated to the background. A doctor walks in, "Who is the nurse for room 310? Can you order ABG stat, PCXR stat, PICC line stat, Foley catheter stat, TPN stat?" and you, "the nurse" trying to be respectful and at the same time, wandering where this self centered doctor was three hours ago when you paged her. No offence to customer service, so you got to take care of business, zip up your mouth and do your function. For sure, she has delayed you while your husband, children and family are waiting for you to prepare dinner, have sex and put them to sleep." NURSES, YOU MOVE ME."

A new doctor came in and asked for the nurse for room 304. The nurse responded and he said, "You need to remove the central line on patient left subclavian." The nurse explained to the doctor that the patient does not have a central line. As they entered the room, the doctor insisted that the patient has a central line. When they got into the patient's room, the nurse demonstrated to the doctor that it is peripheral line (EJ) and not central line. The new doctor thanked the nurse and walked away. EJ Means external jugular. As a nurse, we have contact with doctors more than any other healthcare professional. It is therefore very important for us to have a cordial relationship based on mutual respect and trust. Physicians often think that the only thing nurses do is carrying out their orders. They don't realize that we execute orders that make sense with clarity and no confusion. They do not understand that there is a nursing process which involves Nursing assessment, Nursing diagnosis, planning, intervention and evaluation. Some of the physicians are ignorant of what Nurses do.

The medical diagnoses identify specific pathological problems (Diseases) while nursing diagnoses pinpoint problems that nurses should address and are licensed to treat. That is nursing. Three components for Nursing diagnoses are:

1 The heath problem: What is the health problem? Why is the patient here?

Why was this patient admitted? Why did this client leave his comfort to be here?

2 Signs and symptoms: What signs and symptoms are you as a Registered Nurse able to see by looking and assessing your patient? For example, Diagnoses for cirrhosis for the Liver;

Is the skin and eyes yellowish (jaundice)? What about his abdomen? Is it distended and does patient have ascites? Is there abdominal pain? Is the patient tired and itching most of the time?

What type of cirrhosis? What is the cause, stage and when was it diagnosed?

Confusion, weight loss and muscle wasting. Bilateral leg edema (swelling). The lab result will also guide you. Is your patient confused? Check the ammonia level? Does patient have hepatitis? Abdomen is distended, both legs are swollen this patient should be on a low salt diet.

Another example is pyelonephritis which simply means kidney infection. The kidney is inflamed because of the infection. Your patient has the following:

1 Temperature and chills
2 Pain in the flank, back, groin and abdomen.
3 Complain of pain during urination
4 Frequent urge for urination with small amount each time
5 Smelling, cloudy, miserable-looking urine

This patient for sure needs antibiotic, pain medications, Tylenol or Motrin for temperature, intravenous fluid. This patient will definitely be NPO which means 'Nothing By Mouth.' Patient will also need nephrology consult. Is your patient hypertensive?

Here are some questions for you:

1 What is the relationship between the kidney and hypertension?

2 Renin-angoitensin system. What is the connection with the kidney?

3 Why is this patient NPO? Why is he not fed?

Another funny moment: An eighty-five year old male woke up at 03AM and asked, "Where is my wife?" The nurse replied, "She went home" and the patient replied, "Oh no, she cannot go home. We have been married for sixty-five years." The nurse replied, "she will be back in the morning, go back to sleep." Patient asked, "Where is this place?" Again, Nurse said, "you are in the hospital." The patient responded, "This is hospital. Oh no, this is a hospital? I am dizzy and I think that I am having a heart attack, I am going to die, oh no oh no." After assessing him, we knew that there was nothing wrong with him other than that he was receiving antibiotics for pneumonia and he was demented. The nurse said to patient again, "relax and go back to sleep." The nurse told the patient that his family will visit in the morning but the patient kept saying, "oh no, oh no" followed by snoring. Some for the functions for bedside nursing that are silent include babysitting with lots of tender loving care. Believe it, it is not written anywhere in your contract.

A new nurse with the support from the seasoned nurse placed NGT in the right nare. After the placement, the new nurse went to the charge nurse and told her that NGT was placed and she can please order a Kidney, Ureter and Bladder x-ray to check for placement. The charge nurse looked at her hoping that she will realize her mistake and correct herself but she kept making the same demand. The charge nurse told her that she needed a chest x-ray. The new nurse went to the seasoned Registered Nurse and said to her, "You know what, who made her a charge nurse? She is so stupid. I told her that I needed KUB and she insisted that she will order a chest x-ray to check placement." The seasoned nurse told her that the charge nurse was correct because you would need chest x-ray and not KUB to check for placement. Nasal gastric tube does not go into the kidney, bladder or Ureter, it stops in the stomach. We are having fun, aren't we and you think that we are miserable? The key is to make the best out for it.

Patient has a Foley catheter in place but there was no urine output. The new nurse did not check and see if there was a kink in the tubing, the BUN and

Creatinine or do a bladder scan. She quickly picked up the phone, called the doctor and told the doctor that patient had not voided. The doctor ordered the nurse to put a Foley catheter in and she said to the doctor that the patient has a Foley catheter and the doctor said again to put the Foley catheter in again and the new nurse said, "I will write the doctor up." Most new nurses did not realize that they have accepted employment in one of the most difficult organizational setting in American work force. The Charge Nurse asked what the problem was and she narrated the whole incident to the Charge Nurse and she asked, "Did you check the Foley to see if there is a kink and did you scan the bladder?" and she said, "No." She went and repositioned the patient and fixed the tubing 500ml of cleared color amber rushing into the Foley catheter. You got to know some for these techniques and how to troubleshoot in nursing. Nurses feel powerless in the novice stage of their profession. The biggest challenge is changing from the feeling of powerlessness to empowerment and professionally competent but this is a question of time as long as you are consistently learning, reading, paying attention and hands on procedures. Experience is the best teacher. Experience is not acquired by quitting but by consistency. Patient was hyperventilating "The difficult new nurse" called code blue and immediately called the patient's primary physician for this patient. The doctor ordered the nurse to cancel code blue. She did but went and called Rapid response team (RRT). The doctor was still on the phone with this nurse and told her to encourage her patient to slow down his breathing. The doctor then came in and told the nurse to cancel RRT, gave the patient ice chips and walked away. The new nurse asked, "Why did the doctor look at me like that? Did he think that I am stupid? I am concerned about my patient, that is all." Sometimes, patient demands may become overwhelming for the nurse. Patient is in pain calling every one hour and families making lots for demands and coming to the Nursing Station twenty times in five minutes. The first step in setting your priorities is adequate management of your time.

Evaluate the reason why patient is calling frequently for pain medication. Is the patient under medicated or over medicated? What works for this patient? Does patient have anxiety problem? Is the problem more of anxiety than pain? Find out from the patient or family what works for him. For example, does Norco work better than Percocet? On a scale of zero to ten, with ten been the highest, what is his level of experienced pain? The Charge Nurse for that shift felt humiliated because the new nurse was anxious and powerless and did not comprehend any instructions from anybody. At the end of this case scenario, the nurse burst into tears saying, "God, please I cannot do this, I cannot do this." Both the charge nurse and other nurses reassured her that she can do the job very well. The charge nurse promised her that she will review her assignment and make changes the next day but will help her as much as she could that day.

Is not just the new nurses, some days are like hell even for the seasoned nurses. It is very important for nurses to develop a trustworthy relationship among themselves. Their communication should center on how to provide excellent nursing care. Code blue and RRT were cancelled and this patient was discharged the next day.

CHAPTER FOUR

BULLIES IN THE WORK PLACE

"My dignity may be harassed, assaulted, ridiculed, mocked, and vandalized but it can never be taken away unless I surrendered" Michael J. Fox.

Guess what? Even in nursing, there are bullies. Bullies are not assertive, they are belligerent, truculent, antagonistic, pursuing their aim and interest forcefully, always ready to attack. Bullying can be defined as using threat, force or coercion to abuse, intimidate, or aggressively dominate others. Here is a good example, at 23:00, at the end of my shift, a new admission will be coming and I got report for night shift RN named Roberta, since she refused to get the report herself. I just walked in and I am not ready for Emergency Room report. I have to settle down first. At 23:25, the part-time nursing supervisor called and said that she needed the new man to be transferred to Medical

Oncology. Roberta took the rewritten report to charge nurse and told the charge nurse that I should give report to the new unit. At that point, I refused to do that and told the charge nurse that she should give the report because my time was up. Do the right thing at the right time, and at the right moment. Do not allow bullies to make you make medication errors. Be knowledgeable, know your stuff, read, when in doubt, and ask questions. For example, know the six rights for medication administration; Right patient, route, drug, dose, time and right documentation. "This medication was due in your shift, why didn't you give it? You must give it" she yelled. Please review and make sure that it was not discontinued already.

It can also be referred to as aggressive behavior in which someone intentionally and constantly makes life unbearable for others. There are bullies everywhere; in schools and various other work environments. Bullies should not be tolerated.

27.8% of students, which is nearly one in every three students, were bullied (National center for Education Statistics 2013). Also, 19.6% of high school students in the United States reported being bullied last year in school (Center for Disease Control 2014).

However, we have bullies, that is the way it is. We are one big family with people of various personalities, but with common goals that include patient safety and excellent customer service. Management is entirely aware of the bullying that happens in the workplace, but they consistently fail to address this issue. So many nurses are treated unfairly and the organization fails them, nonunion and union respectively. For example, when organizational rules and policies are violated or employee performance is poor, it is very likely for the institution to see the employee as the problem. The employee becomes discouraged and the trust for the system is drastically reduced. The other solution is to fall back on Equal Employment Opportunity law but be advised as a new nurse that when you go to work, freedom for speech, freedom from searches and the right to assemble are not protected. You can file all your complaints about the bullies, but they all end up nowhere. If the heat is too much, you get out and the bullies stay. You can use the avoidance style by side stepping the problem. This will mean withdrawing from immediate danger without addressing your concern or the concerns of others. You simply have to find a way to live with the bullies. Be safe, take your stand. Nursing is a 24-hour service. But be familiar with what is expected from you in your eight or twelve hours shift. For example, you must check vital signs as ordered, medications should be given, lab must be checked, call doctors for abnormal values, replace what need to be replaced, intake and output must be done, patient acuity, assessment and notes. Do not replace potassium for a dialysis patient ensure you notify the doctor so that it will be taken care of during dialysis.

John Doe is a 46-year old man. He has no medical history, but was found in the parking lot, vomiting blood from his mouth. Intubated by Emergency Medical Technician (EMT), blood alcohol level was 280, left anterior subdural hematoma, left temporal bone fracture. The Magnetic resonance imaging (MRI) conducted on this man showed improvement of SAH, extubated and admitted into Intensive care unit. Alert and oriented X2 stated that he went to a wedding, drank too much, and then he fell. Vital signs stable, condom catheter in place, regular diet, and normal saline levels at 75ml/hr. He does not want to talk to his wife because he they have been separated for 12 years. Nurse called wife on the phone and told her. She came in yelling, "Stupid man, that's why I left, because you're useless and cannot take care of your family or yourself. You homeless bitch, don't ever call my phone again, you fucking bitch" and soon after, she left. You could tell the wife is a bully and probably drove him into drinking. Social workers were notified for placement issue.

CHAPTER FIVE
LEADERSHIP ROLE

In nursing, there are two types of people; leaders and followers. It is important to decide in the beginning of your career whether you want to be a leader or a mere follower. On one hand, it is not a bad idea to be a follower, but there is no credit given when you are a follower. Most great leaders began as great followers because they were able to diligently observe their leaders. Most often in nursing, our desire to be a good leader is often suppressed and kicked to the curb. Do not ask me why, but if you really want to know, you can find the answer in another book. What are the attributes of a good leader?

Qualities of good leaders include:
1. Self control. You have to control yourself, and be able to control others.
2. Self confidence. You must have knowledge, courage, and unwavering honesty based upon ability and knowledge of self.
3. A strong desire for fairness and justice. A fair leader commands respect.
4. Co-operation. A good leader must apply the principle of co-operation and being a great team player.
5. A good leader must have great interpersonal skills and a pleasant personality.
6. Acceptance of full responsibility. A good leader accepts full responsibility of his action and that of his/her followers.
7. Understanding compassion and sympathy. A good leader must have sympathy for his followers.

8. A good leader must have mastery of his leadership position, understand detail of his/her role and function. "Let your light shine before men that they may see your good work and glorify your father which is in heaven." (Matthew 5:16)
9. A good leader has the desire to do more.

In the nursing profession, I encourage everyone to "find their niche." There are various ways you can specialize in a particular field of nursing such as:

Flight Nursing
www.flightweb.com.nursewithoutborders.org
Holistic Nursing: www.indeed.com/Holistic+Nurse
www.ahna.org
Nursing Instructor:registry@yosemite.edu
https//nursesed.net
www.kaplancollege.com
Bedside Nursing: contact Hospitals of your choose County Hospitals/Private Hospitals.

www.ihi.org

Forensic Nursing www.discovernursing.com .

Insurance Nursing:

www.indeed.com/Insurance.com/Insurance+Nurse

Cruise ship Nursing: www.indeed.com/cruise+Ship+Nurse

Hyperbaric Nursing: www.nbdhmt.org

Medical Esthetics Nursing: www.esiw.com

Parish Nursing

:www.parishnurse.orgwww.lifecaremedicalcenter.org

www.nsna.org

Nursing Informatics:

www.himss.orgwww.ushealthonline.com

Traveling Nursing

www.fastaff.com/TravelNursejobs.www.travelnursesourse.com

When you find your niche, stick to it and make the best out of it.

For me, the most interesting and rewarding part of nursing is to work as an instructor in a school. It might probably be because I used to be a high school instructor for so many years. As a college professor (Faculty/Adjunct), you facilitate learning. You motivate, encourage, support, direct and watch them grow in nursing, make mistakes and learn from their mistakes and then drastically improve on it. This is awesome and so fulfilling and in some of the students, you could see yourself, your reaction and attitude when you were a student at twenty-years old.

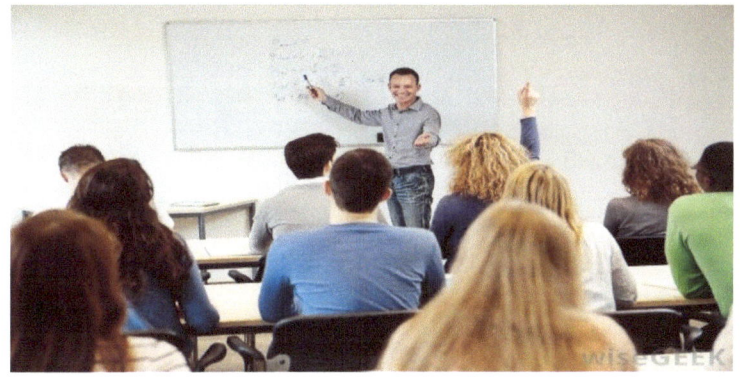

As a nursing instructor, it is your responsibility to participate in assessing the healthcare environments and to be able to predict the trends in nursing education and nursing communication.

You must provide positive ideas to ensure a well-grounded professional workforce for healthcare institutions such as hospitals, companies, school, and insurance companies. Also, provide quality and improve management of students, develop and implement policy and collaborate with hospitals and healthcare providers in the community. It is very exciting to observe new students on the first day during clinical.

The students walk as if they are afraid to show their faces or as if they do not want the patients to see them. Maybe if they walk with confidence, they will break something. Walk like a nurse. Walk with confidence; you have your white coat on and your stethoscope. Go into the patient's room and introduce yourself and tell them who you are and what you can do for them. They know that you are students and most of the patients are happy to see you."

Nursing is a profession of love. A profession that you give yourself to without asking for anything in return. At the beginning of each shift, you do not know what you are going to get. It could be a bad day or a good day. You cannot predict the kind of patient that you are going to get. You do not know whether or not you will be calling a Rapid Response Team or a Code Blue, or a Code Gray during your shift. When you come to work, you pray for the best. But no matter what, you are here and are willing to sacrifice yourself again and again for eight or twelve hours. At the end of your shift, the most important thing that matters is that you have given a piece of yourself to strangers, people that you do not know. You help them no matter how tired your feet are or how badly and unfair they treat you. What is it not to love about nursing? Nursing is full of challenges, problem solving, and troubleshooting. The outfit we wear, our sense of humor; every day, we are learning new things. We surely deal with a lot like hostile patients who spit at us and curse at us but some of these patients turn around to appreciate you and thank you. It is like a family; sometimes, we step into each other's space, and if you have a noncompliance patient, you know that you will be stepping into their space constantly to do a good job if they don't behave. For example, a non-compliant patient decided to smoke in the room with oxygen. You as a Registered Nurse will not allow that because you do not want him to set himself and the room on fire. A female patient had a bowel movement, rang the call light and the nurse came, she said, "I just had bowel movement and it smells really bad. Make sure you wipe me really well, you know I have a big butt."Nurse looked and went to grab a wipe. She went further to say, "I don't like the smell from this room, get some air freshener." The nurse complies with all of her demands but she still was not satisfied. "Who is your manager? You do not show me attitude when I am paying you." The nurse got upset and replied, "you are not paying me, you are homeless and don't even have a job." Patient became quiet but because of her attitude, we quickly transferred her to Med/surgical, as soon as the supervisor made a request for a medical patient to be transferred to another department.

CHAPTER SIX
CONTINUOUS QUALITY IMPROVEMENT

What is CQI: This is a continuous quality improvement.

I have talked about continuous quality improvement (CQI) in the previous chapter but I would like to emphasize on it more. CQI is a work philosophy that supports all the members of an institute or organization to identify new and better ways for implementation of ideas. CQI for healthcare workers means that quality can be improved if backed up by good ideas even if the standard is already high. It is a requirement that all accredited healthcare organization should have quality improvement programs. CQI is growing; it leads to improvement of patient care, a proactive way to improve quality, job satisfaction among healthcare staff. It saves time, which improves a patient's experience. Less time in admission and less discharge waiting time. It reduces stress for patient families and hospital staff. CQI is money saving and cost effective, it reduces misdiagnosis, opportunistic infection, and medication errors.

Workers benefit from CQI. Organizations stand out for excellence. Roles and responsibilities are clearly defined. Communication is more effective and clear. CQI minimizes stress, and healthcare workers adapt to changes more easily and focus on why and how they can make things go well.

In CQI, customers come first. Our number one priority is meeting the expectation and the needs of our customers. The question that arises is "who is your customer?" Customers are external personalities and they include patients and their families, and they are internal when referring to the hospital itself. All workers are encouraged, supported and helped in the improvement of communication among all the departments to be part of the improvement process. Communication should run smoothly among the departments. Nurses should be able to communicate effectively with physicians, physical therapists, or occupational therapists. In accordance to all of these actions, jobs become much more streamlined and get done properly.

How can the CQI work?
There are various model but the steps are the same. But no matter what model that is in place, it is essential to identify important services and the expectation customers have. Customer satisfaction is critical. For example, skin integrity is very important so focusing on prevention of skin breakdown in all high risk areas for bedridden and wheelchair bound patient is very important. The high risk areas include heels, elbows, ears, sacrum/coccyx and over all the bony areas of the body. The steps that should be taken for skin

treatment are; cleaning the skin, then moisturizing the skin, and then protecting the skin.

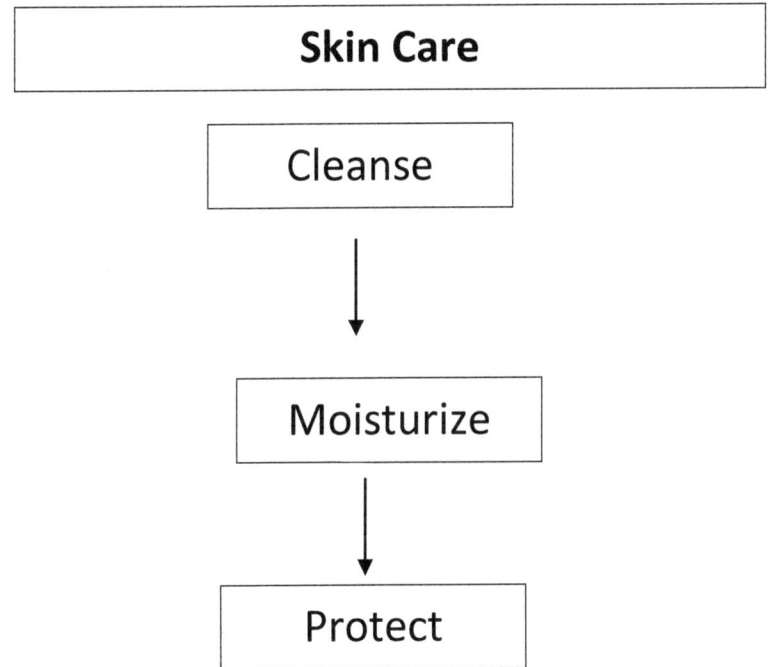

You must work together as a team, no blaming each other, no name calling and no shame. There should be no slow and costly approach to quality, there should be an ongoing process of improvement. Once a new policy is reached, everyone should stick to it. The ideas for quality improvement come from staff who do the work. The responsibility of people at the top is to provide guidance and support in reaching the goal of excellence.

Evaluation of Result

There are several strategies in place for problem solving. Due to a shortage of staff, patients are not re-positioned as often as they should; this often leads to the development of skin breakdown. There should be a meeting between the physician, nurses, physical therapist and occupational therapists to discuss the role of each person in reducing skin breakdown.

Patients should be repositioned every 2 hours and there should be a chart on the wall to show each time that the patient was last repositioned.

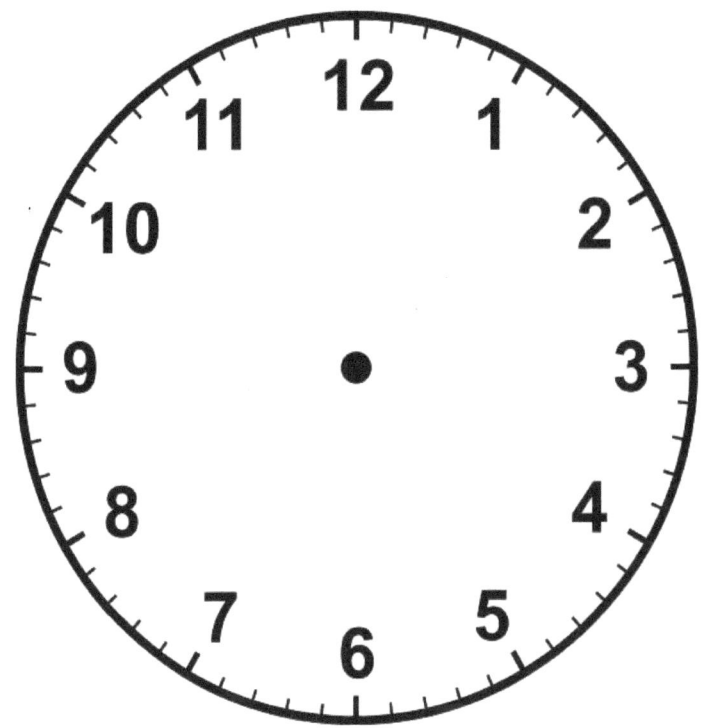

Each individual position should be changed every 2 hours if the patient is bedridden and every one hour if they are in a wheel chair. Patients should be placed in positions to alleviate pressure from bony areas. Being stationary for too long can cause severe discomfort and even clot formation in these patients. For patients that are immobile, their body positioning on a bed with an elevated head will cause them to shift downward. Not only is this not comfortable, but it can make it much harder for such patient to breathe in this position. In general, it is important to assess an individual's mobility so they can be properly monitored and given proper equipment to adjust themselves if possible. Also, you must understand how well your patient can follow directions and if they are able to cooperate. In addition to all this, it is important that these patients eat plenty of healthy food and drink adequate fluids.

Patients should be medicated by the nurse thirty minutes prior to physical activities with a physical therapist to prevent patient from refusing to get out of bed. It is very important for nurses to understand basic skin conditions such as dermatitis, purities, herpes simplex virus, candidiasis, skin tears, venous stasis dermatitis (a form for eczema) xerosis, herpes zoster, scabies exudates, serous, purulent. Also it is important to monitor and prevent skin breakdown. Also to understand Pressure ulcers of various stages from stage 1, stage 11, stage III, stave IV, and unstageable, undermining/tunneling, size and dept ulcers in addition to assessment stages, tunneling and dept for wound. It is important to note odor, pain, duration and foreign body in the wound.

Wounds such as unstageable, stage 111 and stage IV acquired after hospital admissions are reportable by hospitals.

Pressure ulcer care is complex, so you must put in a lot of effort to improve and prevent them. A pressure ulcer develops when something is pressing against the skin and that area of the skin breaks down. A pressure ulcer is also known as a bed sore. It is an injury to the skin and the underlying tissue is the result of that prolonged pressure.

Evaluation of Outcome

Was there a reduction in the number of skin break down? What is the percentage of improvement? Is there a decrease in duration of stay?

The New Ideas

The department has agreed to reposition the patient every two hours and have monitors in the rooms. At the nursing station, the Charge Nurse announced that the manager wanted nurses to use the SBAR during report and also to go to each patient room during report.

Use of SBAR increases effective communication between the nurses and the physician. It makes report to be more friendly and easy.

S: Situation

Here is the situation: Mr. Lopez wound has gotten worse. The wound is now unstageable with slough and eschar.

B: Background

Mr. Lopez developed respiratory failure three weeks ago and was intubated by EMT and was admitted into Intensive Care Unit. In ICU, he was extubated, tracheotomy, and **peg tube placed.** He has a medical history of diabetes, hypertension, back surgery, and total knee replaced one year ago. He was transferred from ICU room to medical/surgery floor five days ago. There was no report of wound to the coccyx area during transfer. The report was that his skin was intact.

A: Assessment

My assessment revealed that patient has wound in the coccyx area and the wound is probably worse than it appears. The patient was not repositioned while in ICU since it was more important to keep him breathing that to look at his buttocks. The wound was developed in ICU but no pictures were taken for appropriate documentation, plan of care, recommendation, evaluation and outcome.

R: Recommendation

I recommend that the doctor should send him to a wound care specialist, have a special bed to be ordered for him, notify the manager, and reposition him every two hours for pressure redistribution and comfort.

Performance improvement is an ongoing process that we continue to improve on what has already been improved.

The Emotional Movements

Philomena,

This is Larry from room 402. I stayed from Jan. 28th to Mar. 31st. My phone number is (262) 222-2222. I still use the mirror that you gave me to shave with. I am taking outpatient physical therapy 3 times a week in the morning. I am walking on my knees now. Thank you very much for everything that you did for me.

Love to see you again,

Larry Fontana

Dear Philomena,

I am not sure if you will remember me, my name is George and I was in room A23. I had burns all over my body and you took good care of me. I refused to eat, but you encouraged me to eat and drink to ensure that I could get my nutrition. Thank you nurse Philomena.

A patient was admitted in room 131A for almost a week. I did not have this patient until his final days on our unit and of his life. I understand that the consequence of life is an inevitable death for every living individual at various stage of life and at different time. But sometimes, some deaths could be very, very painful. Care of a fine young man was delayed due to lack of Health Insurance. Or simply put,

It was delayed because patient was undocumented and was afraid of deportation until his health issue became unbearable.

Isabela: "Nurse, I see you and I know that you know what is wrong with my husband, Joseph. He is not eating and fluid continues to build up in his lungs. Every day, the doctors take out plenty of fluid from his lungs but the doctors say nothing". I will page the doctor for you. As a Registered Nurse, I am not supposed to diagnose but I will page the doctor for you so that they can address your concern. Patient for sure was not doing well. Paged the doctor who gave them the bad news that Joseph has metastatic cancer that has spread. I knew if the Alpha fetal protein (AFP) was elevated, CA 125, CA 19-9 were all high according to the laboratory result. Unfortunately, patient had recently come to United States of America, undocumented and had no job or health Insurance. He was transferred to ICU that night and he died the next day. I cried so much that I was bed side myself. His wife held me and was surprised at my reaction. I encouraged her to be strong and that after the burial of her husband, she must go back to school to be a nurse. I told her that Joseph did not die in vain. His death will bring joy, the impossible will become possible. She did not understand. "Isabela, I said after the burial of Joseph, keep your children with your mother and go back to school." She cried, hugged me tightly and disappeared from the scheme. May God give her strength in a very critical time so that she can move forward. I took a deep breath and calmed myself down. May the soul of Joseph rest in perfect peace. Amen.

REFERENCE:

Wiersema-Bryant LA, BerryJA, Kirby JP. The outpatient wound clinic. In: Krasner DL,ed.chroniC wound care: Essentials.Malvern,PA:HMPcommunication;2014: 331-340

CONCEPTUAL BASES for PROFESSIONAL NURSING Third Edition: Susan Leddy,RN.,PhD.J.B.LIPPINCOTT COMPANY. Phillip J. Decker, PhD

CALCULATE with CONFIDENCE Fourth Edition

Deborah Gray Morris

www.ingramcontent.com/pod-product-compliance
Lightning Source LLC
Chambersburg PA
CBHW040906180526
45159CB00010BA/2951